LOW PROTEIN
DIET FOR
KIDNEY DISEASE

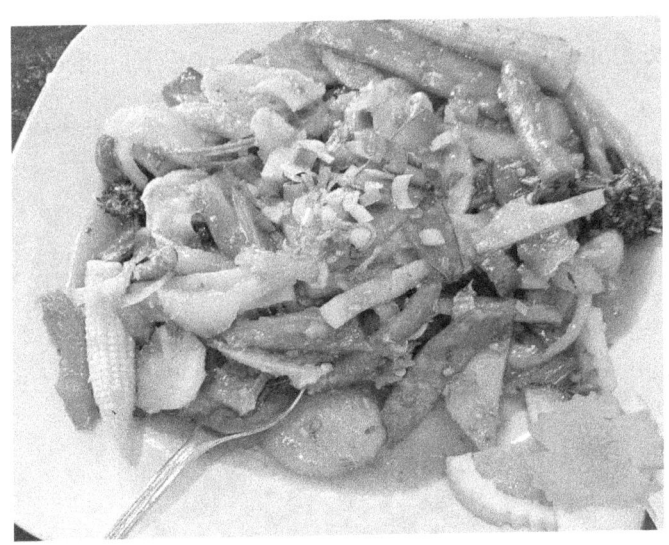

"The Easy guide to Delicious Low-Sodium Recipes to Avoid Dialysis and Manage Chronic Kidney Disease "

Dayna G. Murphy

<u>GAIN ACCESS TO OTHER BOOKS BY ME</u>

TABLE OF CONTENTS

INTRODUCTION

Hook:

In the quiet corridors of healthcare, amidst the hum of fluorescent lights and the beeping of machines, a story unfolds – a story of silent battles fought within the human body. Did you know that over 10% of the global population grapples with the daunting reality of kidney disease? This silent epidemic affects millions, and the battleground is often the dining table. In these pages, we uncover the profound impact of diet on managing kidney disease, revealing the power that lies within every meal to shape the trajectory of one's health.

Personal Connection:

Amidst this widespread health concern, I found myself intimately connected to the journey of kidney disease. Several years ago, a dear friend was diagnosed, and I witnessed firsthand the resilience, sacrifices, and triumphs that define the path of those grappling with this condition. It wasn't just a medical challenge; it was a profound transformation that required a holistic approach to health, particularly in the realm of dietary choices.

Purpose:

Welcome to **"Low Protein Diet for Kidney Disease: A Guide to Navigating Kidney Disease."** In these chapters, our purpose is crystal clear – to be your compass, guiding you through the maze of kidney health with practical, actionable advice. This book is more than just information; it's a lifeline for those seeking not only to understand the intricacies of kidney disease but also to actively take charge of their well-being. We embark on a journey together, exploring the profound connection between diet and kidney health, with a spotlight on the transformative potential of adopting a low protein lifestyle. Are you ready to rewrite your health story? Let's begin.

CHAPTER 1: UNDERSTANDING KIDNEY DISEASE

What is Kidney Disease?

Kidney disease, also known as renal disease, is a progressive condition characterized by the gradual loss of kidney function. The kidneys, vital organs located on either side of the spine, play a crucial role in filtering and removing waste products and excess fluids from the blood. When kidneys fail to function optimally, these waste products accumulate, leading to a range of health complications.

Causes and Risk Factors

Understanding the root causes of kidney disease is pivotal to prevention and management. Explore the diverse factors that contribute to kidney disease, including:

1. Hypertension (High Blood Pressure): Uncontrolled high blood pressure can damage blood vessels in the kidneys over time.

2. Diabetes: Chronic diabetes significantly increases the risk of kidney disease.

3. Genetic Predisposition: Some individuals may have a genetic predisposition to kidney conditions.

4. Autoimmune Disorders: Conditions like lupus and other autoimmune diseases can target the kidneys.

5. Certain Medications: Long-term use of specific medications may contribute to kidney damage.

Stages of Kidney Disease

Kidney disease progresses through stages, each marked by varying degrees of impairment. Understanding these stages is crucial for tailoring effective management strategies. The stages typically include:

1. Stage 1 - *Kidney Damage with Normal or Increased Filtration Rate:* Kidney damage is present, but function remains relatively normal.

2. Stage 2 - *Mildly Reduced Filtration Rate:* Kidney function is mildly impaired, but symptoms may not be apparent.

3. Stage 3 - *Moderately Reduced Filtration Rate:* Kidney function is noticeably reduced, and symptoms may become more apparent.

4. Stage 4 - *Severely Reduced Filtration Rate:* Significant impairment of kidney function, requiring more aggressive management.

5. Stage 5 - *Kidney Failure (End-Stage Renal Disease):* Kidneys are no longer able to function adequately, necessitating dialysis or transplantation.

The Role of Diet in Kidney Health

The relationship between diet and kidney health is profound. Explore the ways in which dietary choices impact the kidneys, including:

1. Fluid Balance: Proper hydration is crucial for kidney function, but excessive fluid intake may strain compromised kidneys.

2. Sodium Intake: Managing sodium levels helps control blood pressure, reducing stress on the kidneys.

3. Protein Consumption: The amount and type of protein consumed can influence kidney function, leading to the exploration of a low protein diet as a therapeutic approach.

Understanding the intricacies of kidney disease sets the foundation for the empowering journey towards kidney health and well-being.

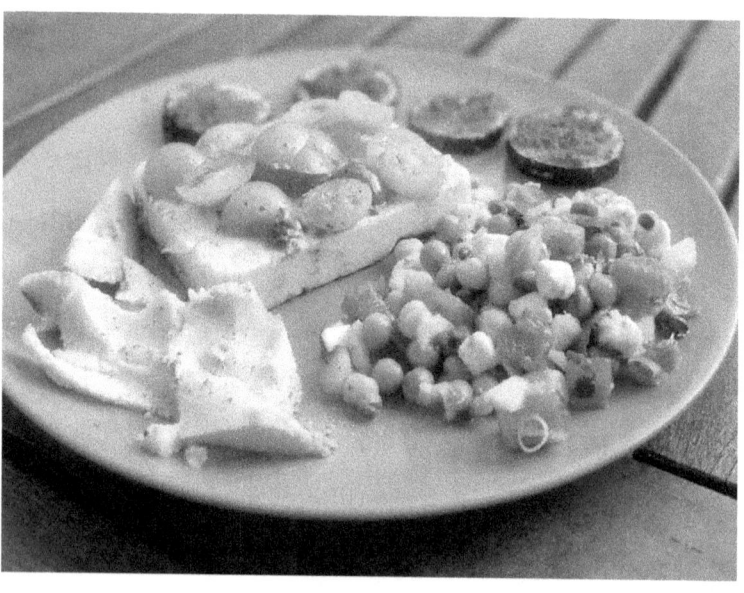

CHAPTER 2: IMPORTANCE OF A LOW PROTEIN DIET

How Protein Affects the Kidneys

Proteins are essential building blocks for the body, but their metabolism generates waste products, including nitrogen. The kidneys play a crucial role in filtering out these waste products. In the context of kidney disease, however, excessive protein intake can exacerbate the strain on compromised kidneys. Explore the mechanisms through which protein affects kidney function:

1. Increased Filtration Load: High protein intake leads to an increased workload for the kidneys, as they must process and eliminate a higher volume of waste products.

2. Impact on Glomerular Filtration Rate (GFR): Excessive protein may contribute to a decline in GFR, a key indicator of kidney function.

3. Proteinuria: Elevated protein levels in the urine (proteinuria) can be indicative of kidney damage.

Balancing Protein Intake

While protein restriction is essential for individuals with kidney disease, it's equally important to strike a balance. Explore strategies for optimizing protein intake while minimizing strain on the kidneys:

1. Quality Over Quantity: Emphasize high-quality protein sources with essential amino acids, such as lean meats, fish, dairy, and plant-based options.

2. Portion Control: Monitor portion sizes to avoid excessive protein consumption.

3. Distributing Protein Intake: Spread protein intake evenly throughout the day to ease the burden on the kidneys.

4. Consultation with a Dietitian: Collaborate with a healthcare professional or dietitian to customize protein recommendations based on individual health status and stage of kidney disease.

Benefits of a Low Protein Diet

A low protein diet tailored to individual needs and kidney function can offer several benefits for those managing kidney disease:

1. **Slowing Disease Progression:** Restricting protein intake may help slow the progression of kidney disease, preserving kidney function.

2. **Reduction of Proteinuria:** A low protein diet can contribute to a decrease in proteinuria, reducing strain on the kidneys.

3. **Blood Pressure Management:** Protein restriction, in conjunction with other dietary measures, can contribute to better blood pressure control, alleviating stress on the kidneys.

4. **Symptom Alleviation:** Some individuals may experience a reduction in symptoms such as edema and fatigue when following a well-managed low protein diet.

By understanding the nuanced impact of protein on kidney function and adopting a balanced approach to protein intake, individuals can harness the benefits of a low protein diet as a valuable tool in their journey towards optimal kidney health.

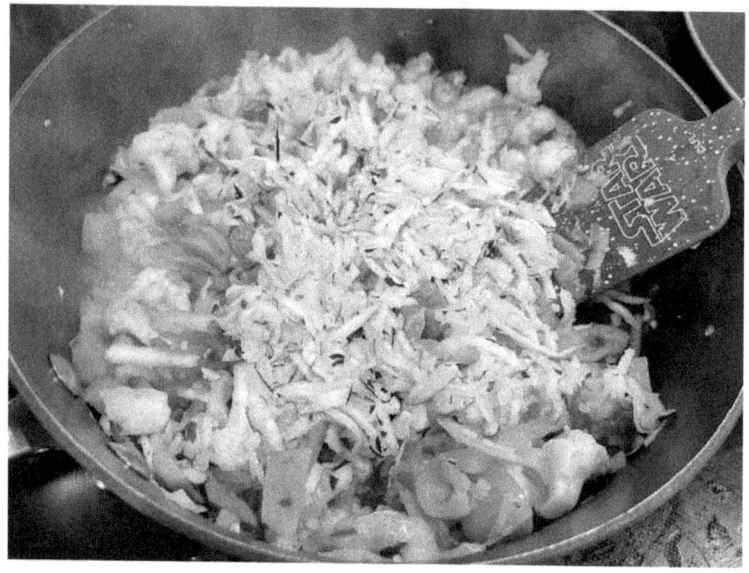

CHAPTER 3: NUTRITIONAL EDUCATION

Essential Nutrients for Kidney Health

While a low protein diet is crucial for managing kidney disease, it's equally important to ensure the intake of essential nutrients that support overall health and kidney function. Explore the following key nutrients and their roles:

1. Potassium: Regulates fluid balance and aids in nerve and muscle cell function. Learn about potassium-rich foods and strategies to manage potassium levels.

2. Phosphorus: Maintains bone health and energy metabolism. Explore sources of phosphorus and methods to control phosphorus intake in the diet.

3. Calcium: Essential for bone health, but its balance with phosphorus is crucial. Discuss dietary sources of calcium and considerations for supplementation.

4. Sodium: Maintaining a controlled sodium intake is vital for managing blood pressure and fluid balance. Understand hidden sources of sodium and strategies for reducing sodium in the diet.

5. Vitamin D: Supports calcium absorption and bone health. Explore ways to ensure adequate vitamin D levels, considering sunlight exposure and dietary sources.

6. Iron and B Vitamins: Addressing specific nutrient needs while considering restrictions imposed by kidney disease.

Supplements and Vitamins

In certain situations, supplements may be recommended to address specific nutrient deficiencies or support overall health. Explore:

1. Iron and Erythropoiesis-Stimulating Agents (ESAs): Discuss the role of iron supplementation in managing anemia associated with kidney disease.

2. Vitamin D and Calcium Supplements: Considerations for supplementing vitamin D and calcium to ensure bone health without overloading the kidneys.

3. B Vitamins: Explore the potential need for B vitamin supplementation and its role in mitigating symptoms associated with kidney disease.

4. Omega-3 Fatty Acids: Discuss the potential benefits of omega-3 supplements in managing inflammation and supporting heart health.

It's crucial for individuals with kidney disease to work closely with healthcare professionals or dietitians to determine specific supplement needs based on their health status and dietary restrictions.

Fluid Intake Guidelines

Optimal fluid management is essential for kidney health, as compromised kidneys may struggle to regulate fluid balance. Discuss:

1. Individualized Fluid Intake Goals: Explore factors such as age, weight, and activity level to determine personalized fluid requirements.

2. Monitoring Fluid Intake: Strategies for tracking daily fluid consumption, considering not only beverages but also foods with high water content.

3. Fluid Restrictions: In certain cases, individuals may need to adhere to fluid restrictions. Understand the reasons for restrictions and methods to stay within recommended limits.

4. Hydration Tips: Practical tips for staying adequately hydrated, including choosing hydrating foods and adjusting fluid intake based on environmental conditions and physical activity.

By providing a comprehensive understanding of essential nutrients, supplements, and fluid management, this chapter equips individuals with the knowledge needed to make informed dietary choices that support kidney health.

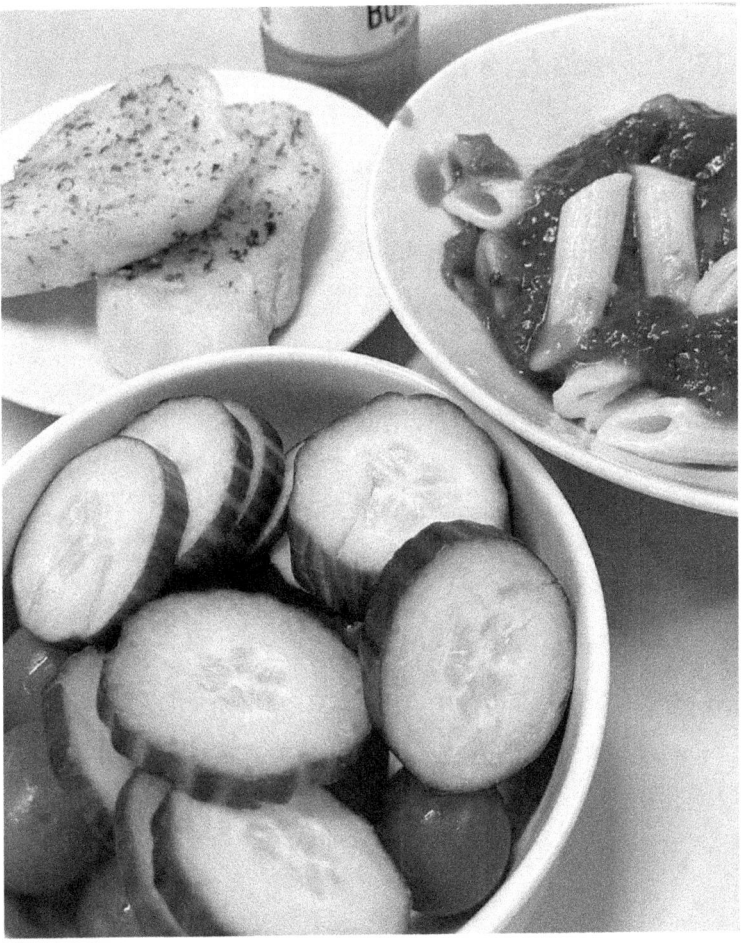

CHAPTER 4: RECIPES IDEAS

Breakfast Recipes

1. Vegetable Omelette

Ingredients:

- 2 eggs
- 1/4 cup bell peppers (diced)
- 1/4 cup tomatoes (diced)
- 1/4 cup spinach (chopped)
- Salt and pepper to taste

Instructions:

- Whisk eggs in a bowl and season with salt and pepper.
- Stir in diced vegetables.
- Pour the mixture into a heated, non-stick pan.
- Cook until the edges set, then flip and cook until fully cooked.
- Serve hot.

2. Greek Yogurt Parfait

Ingredients:

- 1/2 cup low-protein Greek yogurt
- 1/4 cup berries (strawberries, blueberries, or raspberries)
- 2 tablespoons low-protein granola
- 1 tablespoon honey (optional)

Instructions:

- In a glass or bowl, layer Greek yogurt, berries, and granola.
- Repeat the layers.
- Drizzle honey on top if desired.
- Refrigerate before serving.

3. Quinoa Breakfast Bowl

Ingredients:

- 1/2 cup cooked quinoa
- 1/4 cup diced apples
- 1 tablespoon chopped nuts (almonds or walnuts)

- Cinnamon to taste

Instructions:

- Combine cooked quinoa, diced apples, and chopped nuts in a bowl.
- Sprinkle with cinnamon and mix well.
- Microwave for 1-2 minutes or serve cold.

4. Sweet Potato Hash

Ingredients:

- 1 cup sweet potatoes (peeled and grated)
- 1/4 cup onions (diced)
- 1/4 cup red bell pepper (diced)
- 1 tablespoon olive oil
- Salt and pepper to taste

Instructions:

- In a skillet, sauté onions and bell peppers in olive oil until softened.
- Add grated sweet potatoes and cook until tender.
- Season with salt and pepper.
- Serve warm.

5. Cottage Cheese Pancakes

Ingredients:

- 1/2 cup low-protein cottage cheese
- 2 eggs
- 1/4 cup oat flour
- 1/2 teaspoon baking powder

Instructions:

- Blend cottage cheese, eggs, oat flour, and baking powder until smooth.
- Heat a non-stick pan and pour small amounts of batter.
- Cook until bubbles form, then flip and cook the other side.
- Serve with fresh fruit.

6. Avocado Toast with Poached Egg

Ingredients:

- 1 slice low-protein bread
- 1/2 avocado (sliced)
- 1 poached egg

- Salt and pepper to taste

Instructions:

- Toast the bread slice.
- Top with sliced avocado and a poached egg.
- Season with salt and pepper.
- Enjoy immediately.

7. Millet Porridge

Ingredients:

- 1/2 cup millet (rinsed)
- 1 1/2 cups water
- 1/4 cup almond milk
- 1/4 cup diced mango

Instructions:

- Boil millet in water until tender.
- Stir in almond milk and cook until desired consistency.
- Top with diced mango and serve warm.

8. Protein-Packed Smoothie Bowl

Ingredients:

- 1/2 cup low-protein Greek yogurt
- 1/2 cup frozen berries
- 1/2 banana
- 1 tablespoon chia seeds

Instructions:

- Blend Greek yogurt, frozen berries, banana, and chia seeds until smooth.
- Pour into a bowl and add toppings like sliced almonds or fresh berries.

9. Rice Pudding

Ingredients:

- 1/2 cup cooked white rice
- 1/2 cup low-protein milk
- 1 tablespoon raisins
- 1/4 teaspoon vanilla extract

Instructions:

- Combine cooked rice, milk, raisins, and vanilla extract in a saucepan.

- Simmer until thickened.
- Serve warm or chilled.

10. Spinach and Feta Frittata Muffins

Ingredients:

- 4 eggs
- 1/2 cup low-protein feta cheese (crumbled)
- 1 cup fresh spinach (chopped)
- Salt and pepper to taste

Instructions:

- Preheat the oven to 350°F (180°C).
- In a bowl, whisk eggs and stir in feta, spinach, salt, and pepper.
- Pour the mixture into muffin cups.
- Bake for 15-20 minutes or until set.
- Allow to cool slightly before serving.

LUNCH

1. Lemon Herb Grilled Chicken Salad

Ingredients:

- 4 oz boneless, skinless chicken breast
- Mixed salad greens
- Cherry tomatoes, halved
- Cucumber, sliced
- Olive oil, lemon juice, and herbs for dressing

Instructions:

- Season chicken with herbs, grill until cooked.
- Slice and arrange on a bed of salad greens, tomatoes, and cucumber.
- Drizzle with olive oil and lemon juice.

2. Quinoa and Roasted Vegetable Bowl

Ingredients:

- 1/2 cup cooked quinoa
- Roasted vegetables (zucchini, bell peppers, cherry tomatoes)

- Fresh basil leaves
- Balsamic vinaigrette
- Instructions:
- Combine quinoa with roasted vegetables.
- Top with fresh basil leaves and drizzle with balsamic vinaigrette.

3. White Bean and Spinach Soup

Ingredients:

- 1 can white beans (rinsed and drained)
- Fresh spinach leaves
- Low-sodium vegetable broth
- Garlic, onion, and herbs for flavor

Instructions:

- Sauté garlic and onion, add beans and broth.
- Simmer until flavors meld, then stir in fresh spinach.

4. Eggplant and Chickpea Stir-Fry

Ingredients:

- 1 cup diced eggplant
- 1/2 cup chickpeas (canned, rinsed)
- Mixed stir-fry vegetables
- Low-sodium soy sauce

Instructions:

- Stir-fry eggplant, chickpeas, and vegetables.
- Season with low-sodium soy sauce.

5. Salmon and Asparagus Foil Packets

Ingredients:

- 4 oz salmon fillet
- Asparagus spears
- Lemon slices
- Fresh dill

Instructions:

- Place salmon on a foil sheet, surround with asparagus.
- Top with lemon slices and fresh dill, seal into packets.
- Bake until salmon is cooked.

6. Mushroom and Spinach Stuffed Bell Peppers

Ingredients:

- Bell peppers, halved
- Mushrooms, chopped
- Fresh spinach
- Brown rice

Instructions:

- Sauté mushrooms and spinach, mix with cooked brown rice.
- Stuff mixture into halved bell peppers, bake until peppers are tender.

7. Turkey and Vegetable Skewers

Ingredients:

- Turkey breast, cubed
- Cherry tomatoes
- Bell peppers, cut into chunks
- Olive oil, garlic, and herbs

Instructions:

- Thread turkey and vegetables onto skewers.

- Grill until turkey is cooked through.

8. Sweet Potato and Lentil Curry

Ingredients:

- Sweet potatoes, diced
- Red lentils
- Coconut milk
- Curry spices (turmeric, cumin, coriander)

Instructions:

- Cook lentils and sweet potatoes in coconut milk.
- Season with curry spices.

9. Spinach and Goat Cheese Frittata

Ingredients:

- 4 eggs
- Fresh spinach leaves
- Low-protein goat cheese, crumbled
- Cherry tomatoes, halved

Instructions:

- Whisk eggs, mix with spinach, goat cheese, and tomatoes.

- Bake until eggs are set.

10. Cauliflower Rice and Shrimp Stir-Fry

Ingredients:

- Cauliflower rice
- Shrimp, peeled and deveined
- Mixed stir-fry vegetables
- Low-sodium teriyaki sauce

Instructions:

- Stir-fry shrimp and vegetables, add cauliflower rice.
- Drizzle with low-sodium teriyaki sauce.

DINNER

1. Baked Lemon Herb Cod

Ingredients:

- 6 oz cod fillet
- Lemon juice
- Fresh herbs (parsley, dill)
- Olive oil

Instructions:

- Place cod on a baking sheet.
- Drizzle with lemon juice, olive oil, and sprinkle with fresh herbs.
- Bake until the fish is flaky.

2. Lentil and Vegetable Stew

Ingredients:

- 1/2 cup green lentils (rinsed)
- Carrots, celery, and onions (chopped)
- Low-sodium vegetable broth
- Garlic and thyme for flavor

Instructions:

- Sauté garlic, onions, and celery.
- Add lentils, carrots, thyme, and vegetable broth. Simmer until lentils are tender.

3. Chicken and Broccoli Stir-Fry

Ingredients:

- 4 oz chicken breast, sliced
- Broccoli florets
- Low-sodium soy sauce
- Garlic and ginger for flavor

Instructions:

- Stir-fry chicken until cooked.
- Add broccoli, garlic, ginger, and soy sauce. Cook until broccoli is tender.

4. Mediterranean Zucchini Boats

Ingredients:

- Zucchini, halved
- Ground turkey
- Tomatoes, diced
- Feta cheese (low-protein)

- Scoop out zucchini centers.
- Sauté ground turkey and tomatoes, stuff zucchini, and top with feta.
- Bake until zucchini is tender.

5. Shrimp and Avocado Salad

Ingredients:

- 6 oz shrimp, cooked
- Mixed salad greens
- Avocado, sliced
- Balsamic vinaigrette

Instructions:

- Arrange shrimp and avocado on a bed of salad greens.
- Drizzle with balsamic vinaigrette.

6. Tomato Basil Chickpea Pasta

Ingredients:

- Low-protein pasta
- Chickpeas (canned, rinsed)

- Cherry tomatoes, halved
- Fresh basil

Instructions:

- Cook pasta, toss with chickpeas, tomatoes, and fresh basil.

7. Vegetarian Stuffed Bell Peppers

Ingredients:

- Bell peppers, halved
- Quinoa
- Black beans (canned, rinsed)
- Salsa and guacamole for topping

Instructions:

- Cook quinoa, mix with black beans, stuff into bell peppers.
- Bake until peppers are tender.
- Top with salsa and guacamole.

8. Salmon and Asparagus Sheet Pan Dinner

Ingredients:

- 6 oz salmon fillet
- Asparagus spears
- Olive oil, lemon, and herbs for seasoning

Instructions:

- Place salmon and asparagus on a baking sheet.
- Drizzle with olive oil, lemon, and sprinkle with herbs.
- Roast until salmon is cooked and asparagus is tender.

9. Cauliflower and Chickpea Curry

Ingredients:

- Cauliflower, cut into florets
- Chickpeas (canned, rinsed)
- Coconut milk
- Curry spices (coriander, cumin, turmeric)

Instructions:

- Cook cauliflower and chickpeas in coconut milk.

- Season with curry spices.

10. Turkey and Vegetable Skillet

Ingredients:

- Ground turkey
- Mixed vegetables (zucchini, bell peppers, carrots)
- Low-sodium tomato sauce
- Italian herbs for flavor

Instructions:

- Sauté ground turkey, add vegetables and tomato sauce.
- Season with Italian herbs and cook until vegetables are tender.

SNACKS AND APPETIZERS

1. Cucumber and Hummus Bites

Ingredients:

- Cucumber slices
- Hummus (low-protein)
- Cherry tomatoes (optional)

Instructions:

- Spread a small amount of hummus on cucumber slices.
- Top with a halved cherry tomato if desired.

2. Roasted Chickpeas

Ingredients:

- Chickpeas (canned, rinsed)
- Olive oil
- Seasonings (paprika, cumin, garlic powder)

Instructions:

- Toss chickpeas with olive oil and seasonings.
- Roast in the oven until crispy.

3. Stuffed Mushrooms

Ingredients:

- Button mushrooms
- Cream cheese (low-protein)
- Chopped chives

Instructions:

- Remove mushroom stems and stuff with cream cheese.
- Sprinkle with chopped chives.

4. Zucchini Roll-Ups

Ingredients:

- Zucchini strips
- Low-protein ricotta cheese
- Basil leaves

Instructions:

- Spread ricotta on zucchini strips.
- Place a basil leaf on each strip and roll up.

5. Fresh Fruit Skewers

Ingredients:

- Assorted low-potassium fruits (e.g., melons, berries, grapes)

Instructions:

- Thread bite-sized fruit pieces onto skewers.

6. Guacamole and Bell Pepper Slices

Ingredients:

- Bell pepper slices
- Guacamole (low-protein)

Instructions:

- Use bell pepper slices as dippers for guacamole.

7. Cottage Cheese and Pineapple Cups

Ingredients:

- Low-protein cottage cheese
- Pineapple chunks

Instructions:

- Fill small cups with cottage cheese and top with pineapple chunks.

8. Seeded Crackers with Tomato Salsa

Ingredients:
- Low-protein seeded crackers
- Tomato salsa

Instructions:
- Serve seeded crackers with a side of tomato salsa.

9. Edamame Salad Cups

Ingredients:
- Edamame (steamed and shelled)
- Cherry tomatoes, halved
- Balsamic vinaigrette

Instructions:
- Mix edamame and cherry tomatoes, drizzle with balsamic vinaigrette.

10. Fruit Sorbet

Ingredients:

- Low-potassium fruits (e.g., berries, apples)
- Lemon juice
- Sugar substitute (optional)

Instructions:

- Blend fruits, lemon juice, and sugar substitute.
- Freeze for a refreshing sorbet.

BEVERAGES AND SMOOTHIES

1. Berry Blast Smoothie

Ingredients:

- 1/2 cup mixed berries (strawberries, blueberries, raspberries)
- 1/2 banana
- 1/2 cup low-protein yogurt
- Ice cubes

Instructions:

- Blend berries, banana, and yogurt until smooth.
- Add ice cubes and blend again.

2. Cucumber Mint Cooler

Ingredients:

- 1/2 cucumber, peeled and sliced
- Fresh mint leaves
- Lemon juice
- Sugar substitute (optional)
- Sparkling water

Instructions:

- Muddle cucumber slices and mint leaves.
- Add lemon juice, sugar substitute, and top with sparkling water.

3. Pineapple Ginger Refresher

Ingredients:
- 1 cup fresh pineapple chunks
- 1/2 teaspoon grated ginger
- Coconut water

Instructions:
- Blend pineapple and ginger with coconut water.

4. Almond Banana Smoothie

Ingredients:
- 1/2 banana
- 1 cup low-protein almond milk
- 1 tablespoon almond butter
- Ice cubes

Instructions:
- Blend banana, almond milk, and almond butter until creamy.

- Add ice cubes and blend again.

5. Watermelon Mint Fresca

Ingredients:

- 1 cup fresh watermelon cubes
- Fresh mint leaves
- Lime juice
- Water

Instructions:

- Blend watermelon and mint with lime juice.
- Strain and mix with water.

6. Green Tea Lemonade

Ingredients:

- Green tea (brewed and cooled)
- Lemon juice
- Sugar substitute (optional)
- Ice cubes

Instructions:

- Mix green tea, lemon juice, and sugar substitute.

- Serve over ice.

7. Raspberry Coconut Smoothie

Ingredients:
- 1/2 cup raspberries
- 1/2 cup coconut water
- 1/2 cup low-protein coconut milk
- Ice cubes

Instructions:
- Blend raspberries, coconut water, and coconut milk until smooth.
- Add ice cubes and blend again.

8. Strawberry Basil Lemonade

Ingredients:
- 1/2 cup strawberries
- Fresh basil leaves
- Lemon juice
- Sugar substitute (optional)
- Water

Instructions:

- Blend strawberries and basil with lemon juice.
- Mix with water and sweeten if desired.

9. Vanilla Chai Smoothie

Ingredients:

- 1 cup low-protein chai tea (cooled)
- 1/2 teaspoon vanilla extract
- 1/2 banana
- Ice cubes

Instructions:

- Blend chai tea, vanilla extract, and banana until smooth.
- Add ice cubes and blend again.

10. Mango Mint Splash

Ingredients:

- 1 cup fresh mango chunks
- Fresh mint leaves
- Lime juice
- Coconut water

Instructions:

- Blend mango and mint with lime juice.
- Mix with coconut water for a refreshing splash.

DESSERTS

1. Chia Seed Pudding

Ingredients:

- 2 tablespoons chia seeds
- 1/2 cup low-protein almond milk
- 1/2 teaspoon vanilla extract
- Sugar substitute (optional)

Instructions:

- Mix chia seeds, almond milk, and vanilla extract.
- Sweeten with a sugar substitute if desired.
- Refrigerate for a few hours or overnight until it thickens.

2. Baked Apples with Cinnamon

Ingredients:

- Apples, cored and halved
- Cinnamon
- Sugar substitute (optional)

Instructions:

- Place apples on a baking sheet.

- Sprinkle with cinnamon and a sugar substitute if desired.
- Bake until tender.

3. Coconut Lime Sorbet

Ingredients:
- 1 cup low-protein coconut milk
- Lime juice
- Sugar substitute (optional)

Instructions:
- Mix coconut milk with lime juice.
- Sweeten with a sugar substitute if desired.
- Freeze until solid, then blend for a creamy sorbet.

4. Peach and Berry Parfait

Ingredients:
- Low-protein yogurt
- Fresh peaches, diced
- Mixed berries (strawberries, blueberries)
- Granola (low-protein)

Instructions:

- Layer yogurt, peaches, berries, and granola in a glass.

5. Avocado Chocolate Mousse

Ingredients:

- 1 ripe avocado
- 2 tablespoons cocoa powder
- 2 tablespoons honey or sugar substitute

Instructions:

- Blend avocado, cocoa powder, and sweetener until smooth.
- Refrigerate before serving.

6. Almond Flour Cookies

Ingredients:

- 1 cup almond flour
- 2 tablespoons melted butter
- 1/4 cup sugar substitute
- 1/2 teaspoon vanilla extract

Instructions:

- Mix almond flour, melted butter, sugar substitute, and vanilla extract.
- Form into cookies and bake until golden.

7. Berries and Cream

Ingredients:

- Mixed berries (strawberries, blueberries, raspberries)
- Low-protein whipped cream
- Mint leaves for garnish

Instructions:

- Arrange berries in a bowl.
- Top with a dollop of low-protein whipped cream.
- Garnish with mint leaves.

8. Pumpkin Spice Rice Pudding

Ingredients:

- 1/2 cup cooked white rice
- 1/2 cup low-protein milk
- 2 tablespoons canned pumpkin puree
- Pumpkin spice, sugar substitute (optional)

Instructions:

- Combine rice, milk, pumpkin puree, and pumpkin spice.
- Sweeten with a sugar substitute if desired.

9. Lemon Blueberry Frozen Yogurt

Ingredients:

- 1 cup low-protein yogurt
- Zest and juice of 1 lemon
- Blueberries
- Sugar substitute (optional)

Instructions:

- Mix yogurt, lemon zest, lemon juice, and blueberries.
- Sweeten with a sugar substitute if desired.
- Freeze until firm.

10. Strawberry Shortcake Cups

Ingredients:

- Low-protein pound cake, cubed
- Fresh strawberries, sliced

- Low-protein whipped cream

Instructions:

- Layer pound cake cubes, sliced strawberries, and whipped cream in small cups.

CHAPTER 5: LIFESTYLE MODIFICATIONS

Exercise and Physical Activity

Regular exercise is a crucial component of maintaining overall health, and it plays a significant role in supporting kidney health. Engaging in physical activity can contribute to improved cardiovascular function, blood pressure regulation, and metabolic health. However, it's important to tailor exercise routines to individual needs, especially for those managing kidney disease.

Types of Exercise Beneficial for Kidney Health:

1. Aerobic Exercise:

- Activities like walking, cycling, or swimming can enhance cardiovascular fitness and promote overall well-being.

2. Strength Training:

- Building and maintaining muscle strength can help support metabolic health and improve body composition.

3. Flexibility and Balance Exercises:

- Incorporating stretches and balance exercises can enhance mobility and reduce the risk of injury.

Guidelines for Exercise:
- Consult with healthcare professionals or a fitness expert before starting an exercise program, especially for individuals with existing kidney conditions.
- Gradually increase the intensity and duration of exercise to avoid overexertion.
- Stay hydrated and be mindful of fluid restrictions if applicable.

Stress Management Techniques

Stress can have a profound impact on overall health, including kidney health. Chronic stress may contribute to high blood pressure and other conditions that can strain the kidneys. Incorporating stress management techniques into daily life can be beneficial for maintaining both mental and physical well-being.

Effective Stress Management Techniques:

1. Mindfulness Meditation:

- Practicing mindfulness can help reduce stress and promote relaxation. Techniques such as deep breathing and guided meditation can be beneficial.

2. Yoga and Tai Chi:

- These mind-body practices combine physical movement with breath control, promoting relaxation and reducing stress.

3. Regular Physical Activity:

- Exercise releases endorphins, which are natural mood lifters. Engaging in regular physical activity can help manage stress levels.

4. Journaling:

- Writing down thoughts and feelings can provide an outlet for emotions and help individuals gain perspective on stressors.

5. Social Support:

- Maintaining connections with friends and family can provide emotional support and foster a sense of community.

Quality Sleep and its Impact on Kidney Health

Quality sleep is essential for overall health, and it plays a crucial role in supporting kidney function. Chronic sleep deprivation or poor sleep quality can contribute to various health issues, including hypertension and impaired immune function, which can affect kidney health.

Tips for Quality Sleep:

1. Consistent Sleep Schedule:
- Go to bed and wake up at the same time each day to regulate the body's internal clock.

2. Create a Relaxing Bedtime Routine:
- Establish calming pre-sleep rituals, such as reading a book or taking a warm bath, to signal to the body that it's time to wind down.

3. Comfortable Sleep Environment:
- Ensure the bedroom is dark, quiet, and cool. Invest in a comfortable mattress and pillows.

4. Limit Stimulants Before Bed:
- Avoid caffeine and heavy meals close to bedtime, as they can interfere with sleep.

5. Regular Exercise:

- Engaging in regular physical activity can promote better sleep, but it's advisable to avoid vigorous exercise close to bedtime.

6. Manage Stress:

- Incorporate stress management techniques, as chronic stress can disrupt sleep patterns.

7. Limit Screen Time:

- Reduce exposure to screens (phones, computers, TVs) at least an hour before bedtime, as the blue light emitted can interfere with melatonin production.

CONCLUSION

Key Takeaways:

1. Exercise and Physical Activity:

- Engage in a mix of aerobic exercise, strength training, and flexibility exercises.
- Consult with healthcare professionals before starting an exercise program, especially for those managing kidney disease.

2. Stress Management Techniques:

- Practice mindfulness meditation, yoga, or tai chi to reduce stress.
- Regular physical activity is a natural stress-reliever.
- Maintain social connections for emotional support.

3. Quality Sleep and its Impact on Kidney Health:

- Establish a consistent sleep schedule and calming bedtime routine.
- Create a comfortable sleep environment.
- Manage stress and limit stimulants before bedtime.
- Regular exercise can contribute to better sleep.

Encourage Reader Action:

1. Consult Professionals:

- Consult with healthcare professionals or fitness experts before making significant changes to exercise routines, especially for those with kidney conditions.

2. Incorporate Stress Management:

- Integrate stress management techniques into daily life, such as mindfulness practices and regular physical activity.

3. Prioritize Sleep Hygiene:

- Implement good sleep hygiene practices, including a consistent sleep schedule, a calming bedtime routine, and creating a comfortable sleep environment.

Express Hope and Empowerment:

Empower yourself with the knowledge that small, positive changes in lifestyle can have a profound impact on kidney health. By incorporating these practices into your daily routine, you are taking proactive steps toward overall well-being. Remember that each effort, no matter how small, contributes to a healthier and more empowered you. With the right mindset and a commitment to self-care, you can enhance your kidney health and embrace a more fulfilling life. Your journey towards well-being is a journey towards hope and empowerment.

14-DAY MEAL PLAN

WEEK 1

Day 1:

Breakfast: Lemon Herb Grilled Chicken Salad

Lunch: Quinoa and Roasted Vegetable Bowl

Dinner: Baked Lemon Herb Cod

Snack: Roasted Chickpeas

Day 2:

Breakfast: White Bean and Spinach Soup

Lunch: Eggplant and Chickpea Stir-Fry

Dinner: Lentil and Vegetable Stew

Snack: Cucumber and Hummus Bites

Day 3:

Breakfast: Mushroom and Spinach Stuffed Bell Peppers

Lunch: Salmon and Asparagus Foil Packets

Dinner: Chicken and Broccoli Stir-Fry

Snack: Fresh Fruit Skewers

Day 4:

Breakfast: Turkey and Vegetable Skewers

Lunch: Sweet Potato and Lentil Curry

Dinner: Mediterranean Zucchini Boats

Snack: Avocado and Bell Pepper Slices

Day 5:

Breakfast: Spinach and Goat Cheese Frittata

Lunch: Tomato Basil Chickpea Pasta

Dinner: Cauliflower Rice and Shrimp Stir-Fry

Snack: Cottage Cheese and Pineapple Cups

Day 6:

Breakfast: Lemon Blueberry Frozen Yogurt Smoothie

Lunch: Quinoa and Roasted Vegetable Bowl

Dinner: Baked Lemon Herb Cod

Snack: Roasted Chickpeas

Day 7:

Breakfast: Almond Banana Smoothie

Lunch: Lentil and Vegetable Stew

Dinner: Mushroom and Spinach Stuffed Bell Peppers

Snack: Zucchini Roll-Ups

WEEK 2

Day 8:

Breakfast: Lemon Herb Grilled Chicken Salad

Lunch: Quinoa and Roasted Vegetable Bowl

Dinner: Baked Lemon Herb Cod

Snack: Roasted Chickpeas

Day 9:

Breakfast: White Bean and Spinach Soup

Lunch: Eggplant and Chickpea Stir-Fry

Dinner: Lentil and Vegetable Stew

Snack: Cucumber and Hummus Bites

Day 10:

Breakfast: Mushroom and Spinach Stuffed Bell Peppers

Lunch: Salmon and Asparagus Foil Packets

Dinner: Chicken and Broccoli Stir-Fry

Snack: Fresh Fruit Skewers

Day 11:

Breakfast: Turkey and Vegetable Skewers

Lunch: Sweet Potato and Lentil Curry

Dinner: Mediterranean Zucchini Boats

Snack: Avocado and Bell Pepper Slices

Day 12:

Breakfast: Spinach and Goat Cheese Frittata

Lunch: Tomato Basil Chickpea Pasta

Dinner: Cauliflower Rice and Shrimp Stir-Fry

Snack: Cottage Cheese and Pineapple Cups

Day 13:

Breakfast: Lemon Blueberry Frozen Yogurt Smoothie

Lunch: Quinoa and Roasted Vegetable Bowl

Dinner: Baked Lemon Herb Cod

Snack: Roasted Chickpeas

Day 14:

Breakfast: Almond Banana Smoothie

Lunch: Lentil and Vegetable Stew

Dinner: Mushroom and Spinach Stuffed Bell Peppers

Snack: Zucchini Roll-Ups